Edward Hitchcock

A Manual of the Gymnastic Exercises

As Practised by the Junior Class in Amherst College, Amherst, Mass

Edward Hitchcock

A Manual of the Gymnastic Exercises
As Practised by the Junior Class in Amherst College, Amherst, Mass

ISBN/EAN: 9783337178635

Printed in Europe, USA, Canada, Australia, Japan

Cover: Foto ©Andreas Hilbeck / pixelio.de

More available books at **www.hansebooks.com**

OF THE

GYMNASTIC EXERCISES

AS PRACTISED BY

THE JUNIOR CLASS IN AMHERST COLLEGE

AMHERST, MASS.

PREPARED UNDER THE DIRECTION OF

DR. EDWARD HITCHCOCK

PROFESSOR OF PHYSICAL EDUCATION AND HYGIENE

BOSTON

PUBLISHED BY GINN, HEATH, & COMPANY

1884

INTRODUCTION.

THE need of a manual like the present is seen in the fact that three editions of a similar work have been issued at Amherst during the past few years. The recent advances made in this department, and the increased facilities of our new Pratt Gymnasium, now ready for occupancy, seem to demand a new manual, and one which shall more fully meet the practical wants of teachers and educational institutions everywhere.

The object of this manual is to furnish a series of exercises, by the use of which a teacher can directly instruct a class in light gymnastics; or an ingenious person may take the leading points in these exercises, and adapt them to peculiar wants and circumstances, thus giving a greater variety and pleasure of movement.

There is also given a series of simple military movements that may be made by a class or company of from twenty to a hundred, — male or female, — either in a small out-of-doors area, or in an ordinary hall.

Persons who may wish either to direct themselves or others to a special use of certain parts of the body, and to learn what muscles are used in different exercises, will find a portion of the manual devoted to this use: it is not claimed, however, that every muscle used in each of these exercises is clearly stated here. Most movements of the body are too complex to allow of perfect specialization in so short a work as this.

Two tables are given, showing certain measurements of the human body. One is made from several thousand measurements of twenty-one hundred and six students of Amherst College, covering an interval of twenty years, and expressed in the ordinary English system of measures. The other is made from measurements of four hundred and sixty-one students, comprising more than fifty different data, covering a space of three years, and expressed in the metric system.

The dumb-bell exercise was devised and first given by Professor E. Hitchcock, jun., of Cornell University; but the preparation of it in a written form, as well as of the marching movements, has been most carefully made by Mr. Frank E. Whitman, the captain of '85. The study of the muscles used in the dumb-bell movements has been made by Mr. C. H. Nichols of the same class, and the cuts have been designed by Mr. H. M. Waite of the class of '85. All the exercises — bells and marching — are executed by the present senior class, or the class of '85.

A schedule for marking the different movements and exercises in a gymnastic exhibition is given directly after the tables. In its present form, it supposes at least three classes in competition for a prize, and the contest to consist of marching movements and a dumb-bell exercise. It also supposes that the dumb-bell exercise shall receive one mark, while each one of the several marching movements is to be graded by the maximum as expressed in the printed number against each movement.

EDWARD HITCHCOCK,

Professor of Hygiene and Physical Education,
AMHERST COLLEGE.

MANUAL

OF

GYMNASTIC EXERCISES.

MARCHING EXERCISE.

In the following instructions for the drills in marching and light gymnastics as practised in Amherst College, an attempt has been made to describe the various movements in the manner best suited for the use of the gymnasium. It will, on this account, be noticeable to any one versed in military tactics, that many deviations have been made from the instructions as laid down in " Upton's Infantry Tactics," or as taught in the military schools. In the main, however, the marching movements here given are taken, with only slight changes, from " Upton's Infantry Tactics ; " and many of the instructions are given just as they appear in that book.

1. **The Arrangement of the Gymnasium.** — In order that the class may have ample room for the dumb-bell exercise, and particularly for marching, the apparatus for heavy gymnastics should be arranged, as far as practicable, on the sides and at the back of the hall. A platform for the pianist and captain should be placed in the front of the hall. For holding the bells when not in use, hooks may be arranged in a row around the hall, at about five feet

from the floor; or boxes may be placed at convenient points, so that the men may take and leave their bells as they file around the hall.

2. The Dumb-bell. — The dumb-bell should be turned out of well-seasoned, first-quality rock-maple, and measure ten inches in length; the balls being three inches in diameter, and the handle measuring four by one and one-fourth inches. Such a dumb-bell weighs one and one-fourth pounds, and may be considered too light; but a heavier one has been found to be unwieldy, and too fatiguing for a briskly performed exercise.

3. The Uniform. — It has been found very convenient, in fact almost necessary, for the classes to have some kind of uniform for gymnasium practice. The uniform that has given most satisfaction in Amherst consists of a loose-fitting shirt and a pair of trousers, both of dark-blue Middlesex flannel. The shirts are usually made to button on the shoulder, so as to leave the breast clear for a class or college monogram. The trousers are of the style commonly known as " hip-pants."

4. Arrangement of Classes into Platoons. — Classes numbering more than thirty men should be divided into platoons, and each of these placed in charge of a " platoon captain," whose duty it is to see that the class movements are properly executed, and to give such orders as are indicated in the instructions. A platoon should consist of not less than three nor more than six fours. It will be noticed, that in the marching movements, as arranged for the gymnasium, there is no such thing as " double rank."

5. Music and Time. — In theory, the time occupied by the motions in the dumb-bell exercise is nothing, the body and bells being at rest all the time; and in practice, we must come as near to this as possible, — that is, the motions must be made very rapidly. The time of the music may vary, and with it will vary also the periods of rest between the counts ; but the rapidity of the movements should be always the same.

Galop or march music may be used, and hence the term "count" has been employed instead of "beat."

The phrase "through —— counts " may seem ambiguous in some places. It invariably means, till —— counts have been completed.

6. **Commands.** — Commands are of two kinds, — the *preparatory command*, such as *Forward*, which indicates the movement that is to be executed ; the command of *execution*, such as MARCH, HALT, which causes the execution of a command. In the following instructions, the preparatory commands are distinguished by *italics*, and those of execution by SMALL CAPITALS.

The tone of command is animated, distinct, and of a loudness proportioned to the number of men under instruction.

Each preparatory command is pronounced in an ascending tone of voice, and always in such a manner that the command of execution may be more energetic and elevated.

The command of execution is pronounced in a tone firm and brief.

7. **Assembling the Class.** — At the captain's command, *Fall* — IN, each platoon takes its proper position in a column of files ; i.e., in "single file," following the captain as he marches around the hall. The men must keep their heads and eyes directly to the front, must cover the men in front of them, and keep closed to the *facing distance;* that is, such a distance, that, in forming into line,

the elbows will just touch. The arms should hang naturally at the sides, without stiffness, but without swinging. The full step is twenty-eight inches in length, measuring from heel to heel; and the cadence for marching in the gymnasium should be ninety steps per minute.

8. **To bring the Platoons on Line.** — At the captain's command, *On line* — MARCH, the platoon captains take command of their platoons, and, by repeating the above order, bring their platoons to their respective places.

9. **To arrest the March.** — The command is, *Platoon* — HALT. At the word *Halt*, given the instant either foot is brought to the ground, the foot in the rear is brought up, and planted by the side of the other without shock.

10. **Facings.** — The command is, *Left* (or *Right*) — FACE. At the word *Face*, raise the right foot slightly, face to the left (or right), turning on the left heel, the left toe slightly raised; replace the right heel by the side of the left, and on the same line. If the proper *facing distance* was kept in marching, it will be found that the elbows just touch. It will be seen that the facings to the right or left are both made on the *left* foot.

11. **Alignment.** — The platoon captains place themselves at the heads of their respective platoons, facing down the line, and command, *Right* — DRESS. At the command *Dress*, every man turns the head and eyes sharply to the right, so that he can see the breast of the second man from him; then, without inclining the head, he takes very short steps, either backward or forward, or to the left if the line is crowded, but never *crowding* toward the *right* until the line is perfected, when the platoon captain commands FRONT, at which word every head turns sharply to the front.

The class captain then commands, *Company — Right Dress* — FRONT, at which the entire class repeats the above.

12. **The Position.** — The men should now be occupying the following position : After effecting an equal squareness of the body and shoulders to the front, place the heels well closed on the same line, with the knees straight, and the feet forming an angle of about sixty degrees.

Let the arms hang naturally, slightly turning at the elbows, with the palms of the hands turned slightly to the front, and the little fingers touching the seams of the trousers, the thumb and forefinger closed.

Hold the body erect on the hips, inclining it sufficiently forward to cause its weight to principally bear upon the fore-part of the feet.

Hold the head erect, with the eyes straight to the front.

13. **The Salute.** — The command is, *Company — SALUTE.* At the word *Salute*, (1) raise the right hand smartly, pointing in the same direction as the right foot, the palm of the hand down, the thumb close to the forefinger, the arm extended and horizontal ; (2) bring the hand around till the point of the thumb and side of the forefinger touch the forehead ; (3) bring back the hand and arm to the position of the first motion ; (4) drop the arm quickly by the side.

14. **To count Fours.** — The command is, *Count — FOURS*; at which each platoon, beginning on the right, counts 1, 2, 3, 4. 1, 2, 3, 4, etc., through the platoon.

The class is now ready for either the dumb-bell exercise or the marching movements. If it is desired to take the former, the captain commands, *Offset — MARCH.* At the word *March*, man number one remains where he is ; number two takes two paces to the front, and stands on the V in front of him; number three takes four paces, and number four takes six paces, occupying their respective Vs. This will be made clear by a glance at the floor diagram, Fig. 1.

If, however, it is desired to take the marching movements, the class should be made

15. To form Column of Files from Column of Platoons. — The command is, *By Platoons* — *By the Right Flank* — MARCH. At the word *March*, the platoon which is in front is commanded by its captain, *Right* — FACE. This is described in Section 9. At the command, *Forward* — MARCH, the platoon, now in a column of files. marches promptly with the full step. The other platoons are commanded by their captains, *Forward* — *Guide Right* —MARCH ; care being taken, however, to wait long enough to avoid colliding with the platoon next in front. At the word *March*, the men step off smartly with the left foot : the guide (i.e., the man on the extreme right of each platoon) marching straight to the front. It must be observed, in marching thus, that the men touch lightly the elbow toward the side of the guide ; that they open out neither arm ; that they yield to pressure coming from the side of the guide, and resist pressure coming from the opposite direction ; that, shortening or lengthening the step, they gradually recover the alignment and touch of the elbow, if lost ; and that they keep the head direct to the front.

When the platoon reaches the front of the hall, the captain commands, *By the Right Flank* — MARCH. At the word *March*, given as the right foot strikes the floor, advance and plant the left foot, then turn to the right, and step off in the new direction with the right foot. If it is desired to flank to the *left*, give the word *March* as

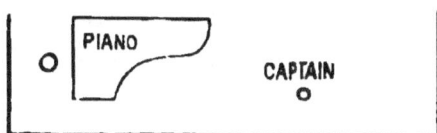

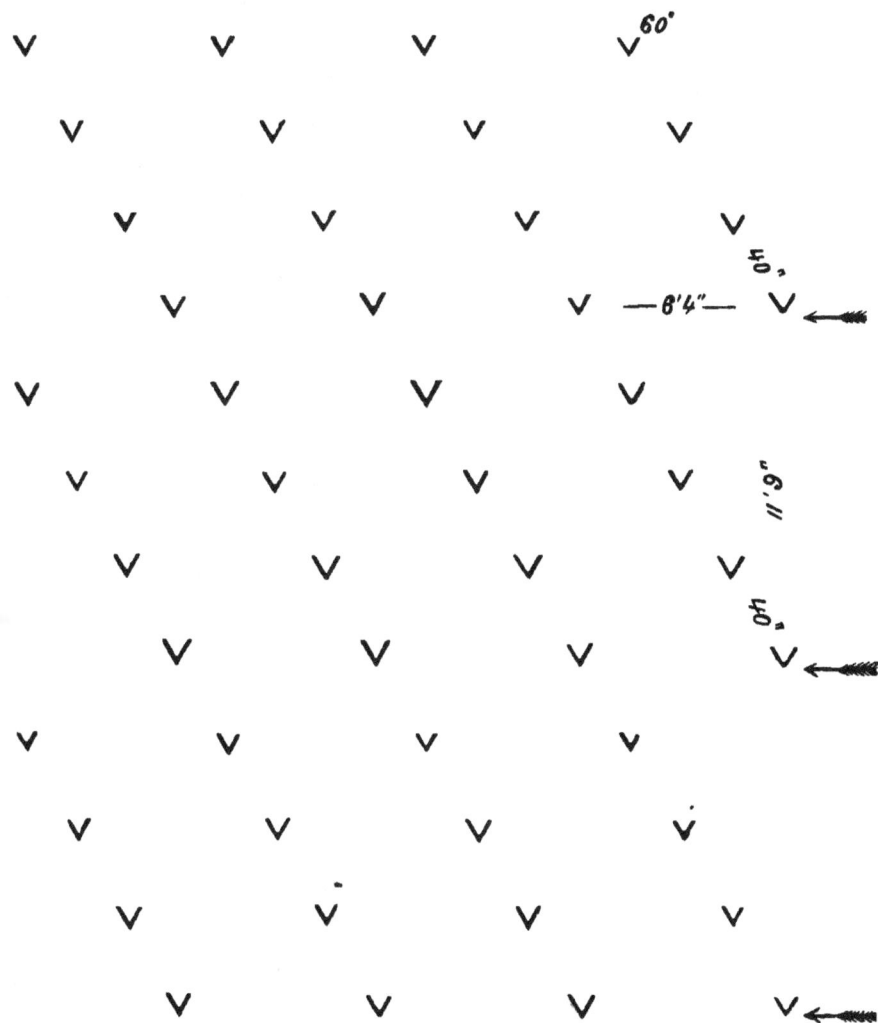

Fig. 1.

the *left* foot strikes the floor, advance and plant the right foot, turn to the left, and step off in the new direction with the *left* foot.

When all the platoons have executed this movement, the class will be marching around the hall in a column of files.

The movements from Section 15 to Section 21, inclusive, are executed at the class captain's command.

16. **To form Column of Two from Column of Files.** — The command is, *Form Twos — Left Oblique — March.* At the word *March*, numbers one and three take the short step, numbers two and four oblique to the left until they uncover the men in front of them, when they resume the forward march; the twos having united, all resume the full step. It will be observed, that the distance between the twos remains the same as it was between numbers *one* and *three*. [Fig. 2.]

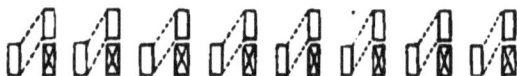

Fig. 2.

17. **To form Column of Fours from Column of Twos.** — The command is, *Form Fours — Left Oblique — March.* At the word *March*, the leading two of each four take the short step; the rear two oblique to the left until they uncover the leading two, when they resume the forward march; the fours having united, all resume the full step. It will be observed, that the distance between the fours is twice the distance between the twos; in fact, the space between the fours should be a square.

18. **To shorten the Step.** — The command is, *Short Step — March.* At the word *March*, the length of the

step is reduced to fourteen inches; the class resuming the full step at the command, *Forward* — MARCH.

19. **To change Step.** — The command is, *Change Step* — MARCH. At the word *March*, given the instant the right foot comes to the floor, the left foot is advanced and planted; the hollow of the right is then advanced against the heel of the left, the man again stepping off with the left.

20. **To march to the Rear.** — The command is, *To the Rear* — MARCH. At the word *March*, given as the right foot strikes the floor, advance and plant the left foot; then turn on the balls of both feet toward the right, and immediately step off with the left foot.

21. **To mark Time.** — The command is, *Mark Time* — MARCH. At the word *March*, given the instant one foot is coming to the ground, continue the cadence, and make a semblance of marching, without gaining ground, by alternately advancing each foot about half its length, and bringing it back on a line with the other.

At the command, HALT, given as either foot comes to the floor, plant that foot, and bring the other to its side.

The class resumes the march at the command, *Forward* — MARCH.

22. **To march Column of Fours in Retreat.** — The command is, *Fours Left* (or *Right*) *About* — MARCH. The fours wheel on a fixed pivot: i. e., the pivot-man, number four, in *Fours Left About*, simply marks time in his place, turning his body as the four turns; the flank man, number one, in *Fours Left About*, takes the full step, describing a semicircle to the left; the other men in the four turning with him, and accommodating their step to their position in the four. When the fours have completed a semicircle, all, thus faced directly to the rear,

step off with the full step in the new direction. In executing movements similar to this, in order to preserve the alignment of the fours, the flank-man casts his eyes toward the pivot-man, and feels lightly the elbow of the next man toward the pivot, but never pushes him. The other men touch with the elbow toward the pivot, and resist pressure from the opposite side.

The movements from Section 22 to 28, inclusive, are executed at the command of the *platoon captains*, who take the command from the class captain.

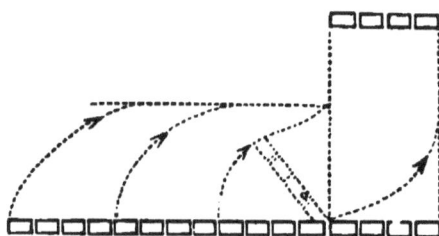

Fig. 3.

23. To oblique in Column of Fours. — The command is, *Left* (or *Right*) *Oblique* — MARCH. At the command, *March*, every man faces one-half to the left, and marches with the full step in that direction, resuming the forward march at the command, *Forward* — MARCH. During the oblique, the fours preserve their parallelism; the man in each four, on the side toward which the oblique is made, is the guide of the rank. [Fig. 4.]

24. To form Column of Platoons from Column of Fours. — The command is, (1) *Left Front into Line* — (2) MARCH; (3) *Platoon* — (4) HALT; (5) *Right* — (6) DRESS — (7) FRONT. At the command, *March*, the first four moves straight to the front, dressing to the right; the other fours oblique to the left, till opposite their places in the line, when each marches to the front. At the command, HALT, the first four halts, and at the sixth command, given immediately after, dresses to the right; the other fours halt, dressing to the right on arriving in line: the seventh command is given when the last four completes its dressing. As each four arrives in line, the men must be careful not to overstep the line, but to halt *together* a few inches in the rear of the line. [Fig. 5.]

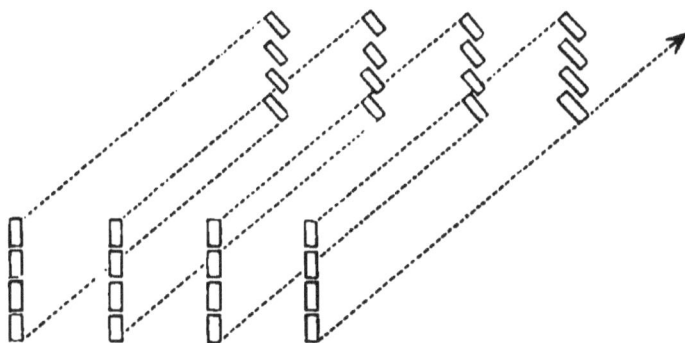

FIG. 4.

25. **To break into Column of Fours.** — The command is *Right Forward, Fours Right* — MARCH. At the command, *March*, the right four moves straight to the front, shortening the first three or four steps; the other fours wheel to the right, on a fixed pivot; the second four, when its wheel is two-thirds completed, wheels to the left on a movable pivot, and follows the first four; the other fours, having wheeled to the right, move forward, and wheel to the left on a movable pivot, on the same ground as the second. [See Fig. 3.]

The difference between wheeling on a fixed pivot and wheeling on a movable pivot is, that in the former the pivot-man simply marks time in his place, turning in conformity with the marching flank, and making no headway; while, in wheeling on a movable pivot, the pivot-man

takes short steps of nine inches, turning in conformity
with the marching flank, and making slight headway.

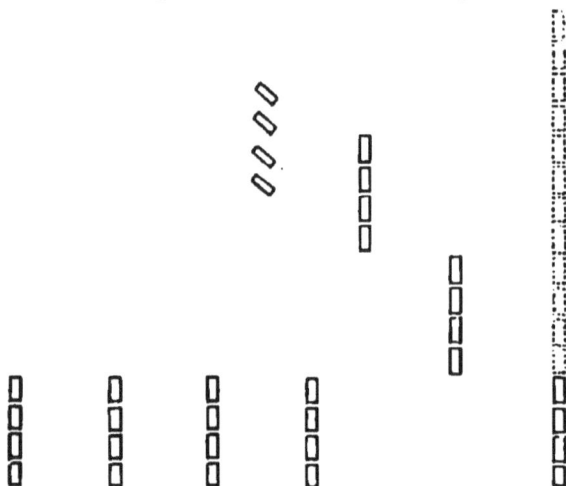

FIG. 5.

26. **To flank to the Front, from Column of
Fours.** — The command is, *Fours Left* (*or Right*) —
MARCH.   At the command, *March*, the fours wheel to the
left, on a fixed pivot.   The platoon captain commands
Guide — RIGHT (or LEFT), the instant the fours unite in
line.   The instructions for *Guide Right*, and for marching
in line across the floor, are given in Section 14.   When
the platoon reaches the front of the hall, if it is desired
to break into a column of fours, the command is, *Right
Forward, Fours Right* — MARCH.   This is described in
Section 24.   If it is desired to break into a column of
files, the command is, *By the Right Flank* — MARCH.   This
is described in Section 14.

27. **To flank to the Front from Column of Files.**
— Considering that the last command was, *By the Right
Flank*, and the class thus formed into a column of files,
the command for this movement is, *By the Left Flank* —

March. This is described in Section 14. On reaching the front of the hall, either command suggested in Section 25 may be used.

28. **To form Column of Twos from Column of Files.** — See Section 15.

This completes the marching-drill as practised at the exhibition in Amherst College. There may be occasions when it will be convenient to use a few movements which are not given in the foregoing instructions for the marching-drill. A few of these movements are thus described :

29. **To march to the Side.** — Being at a halt, the command is, *Side Step to the Right* (or *Left*) — March. At the command, *March*, carry the right foot six inches to the right, keeping the knees straight and the shoulders square to the front ; as soon as the right foot is planted, bring the left foot to the side of it, and continue the movement, observing the cadence, until the command, Halt.

30. **To march Backward.** — Being at a halt, the command is *Backward -- Guide Right* (or *Left*) — March. At the command, *March*, step off smartly, with the left foot, fourteen inches straight to the rear, measuring from heel to heel. At the command, Halt, bring back the foot in front to the side of the one in the rear.

31. **To form Column of Twos from Column of Fours.** — The command is, *Right by Twos* — March. At the command, *March*, the two men on the left of the four (i.e., numbers three and four) mark time for an instant, till they become disengaged, when they oblique to the right, and take their positions behind numbers one and two.

32. **To form Column of Files from Column of Twos.** — This is executed in precisely the same manner as Section 30 ; the command being, *Right by File* — March.

The following schedule will show the relative importance attached to the different movements, and also the order usually pursued.

MARKING SCHEDULE FOR GYMNASTIC EXHIBITION.

COMPANY MOVEMENTS.	Maxima.	Freshmen.	Sophomores.	Juniors.
1. To form columns of twos . .	3			
2. To form columns of fours . .	3			
3. Short step	3			
4. Change step	3			
5. To the rear	5			
6. Mark time, halt	3			
7. To march column of four in retreat	10			
8. To oblique in column of fours (by platoons)	10		•	
9. To form platoons (left front into line)	10			
10. To break into column of fours .	5			
11. To flank to front from column of fours	10			
12. To break into column of files .	5			
13. To flank to front from column of files	10			
14. To form column of twos and leave the hall	5			
15. { Steadiness, Distances, }	15			
Dumb-bell exercise	100			
Totals				
Average				

THE DUMB-BELL EXERCISE.

After the men have taken their positions on Vs, at the command, *Offset* — MARCH, the captain commands, *Bells* — READY. At the word "Ready," the bells are brought instantly and noiselessly to the sides, where they are held horizontal and parallel to each other. At the command, BEGIN, the class begins the following exercise. accompanied by the pianist.[1]

Movement 1. DIRECTION A. — Forcibly twist both bells inward, and back again to position, on each count. through six counts; on seven, carry the bells to the breast, just in front of the armpits; on eight, extend the arms horizontally forward, bells perpendicular, when the men will be in position for

DIRECTION B. — Twist bells as in A, through six counts; on seven, carry bells to the breast; on eight. extend arms horizontally at sides, bells perpendicular, the position for

DIRECTION C. — Twist bells as in A, through six counts; on seven, carry bells to the shoulders; on eight. extend arms perpendicularly, bells horizontal, the position for

DIRECTION D. — Twist bells as in A, through six counts : on seven, carry bells to the breast, and rest there through count eight.

Movement 2. DIRECTION A. — Forcibly thrust the

---

[1] For the arrangement of the class for dumb-bell exercise, consult page 5 *et seq.*

right bell forward horizontally on count one, and return to breast on two, continuing thus through eight counts.

Same with left bell, through eight counts.

On count one, forcibly thrust the right bell forward horizontally, and return on count two; on count three, thrust left bell forward in same manner, and return it to breast on count four; continuing thus alternately through eight counts.

Forcibly thrust *both* bells forward simultaneously, through eight counts.

DIRECTION B. — Repeat all the movements of A horizontally outwards.

DIRECTION C. — Repeat all the movements of A perpendicularly upwards.

DIRECTION D. — Repeat all the movements of A vertically downwards.

Movement 3. — The bells being at the breast, parallel to each other, on count one forcibly thrust the right bell vertically upwards and the left bell vertically downwards; on count two, return both bells to the breast; on count three, thrust the left bell upward and the right downwards, returning to breast on count four, and so continue through twelve counts.

Movement 4. — Both bells being at the breast on count twelve, on count one extend both bells horizontally outwards, bells perpendicular, and hold them thus through four counts.

Movement 5. DIRECTION A. — Drop the arms, without bending the elbows, so that the bells strike just in front of the body, on the ends toward the little fingers; on count two, turn the bells, and strike the ends toward the thumbs; continuing thus through twelve counts. [Fig. 6.]

DIRECTION B. — Same as A, but striking just behind the body, through twelve counts.

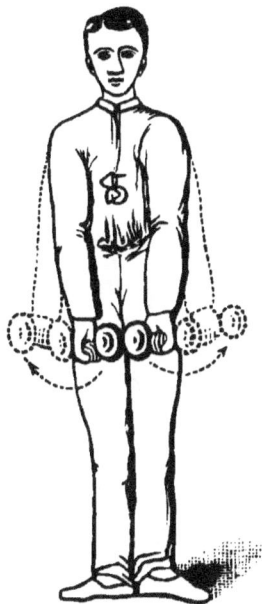

FIG. 6.

DIRECTION C. — On count one, strike bells just in front of the body, ends toward little fingers together; on count two, strike just behind the body, ends toward thumbs together; and continue thus through twelve counts.

DIRECTION D. — On count one, strike the bells just in front of the body, ends toward little fingers together, as before; on count two, strike behind; on three, in front again; on count four, let the bells describe a semicircle outwards, and strike above the head on ends toward thumbs; continuing thus through twelve counts

Movement 6. DIRECTION A. — The bells being above the head on count twelve, on count one advance the right

foot, with a stamp, about four inches in the direction of
the right arm of the V; separate the bells slightly, about
six inches, and strike them on the ends toward the
thumbs, at the same time the step is taken; continue
the step and stroke through four counts. The right knee

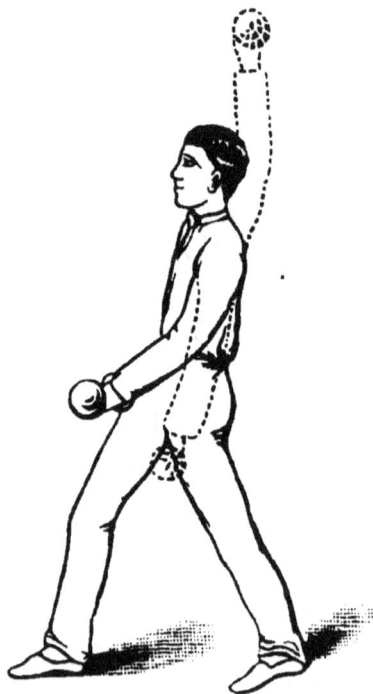

Fig. 7.

being slightly bent, at count one strike the bells together
— ends toward little fingers — just above the leg; on
count two, strike ends toward thumbs together just beneath the leg; on count three, strike ends toward thumbs
together above the head; and continue thus through
twelve counts. Recover the regular position by drawing
the foot back four inches each count, through four counts,
striking the bells above the head as in making the charge.

DIRECTION B. — Repeat A toward the left.

Caution. — Bend the back but *slightly* in striking beneath the leg.

Movement 7. — After recovering from the charge to the left, the bells are above the head on count four. On

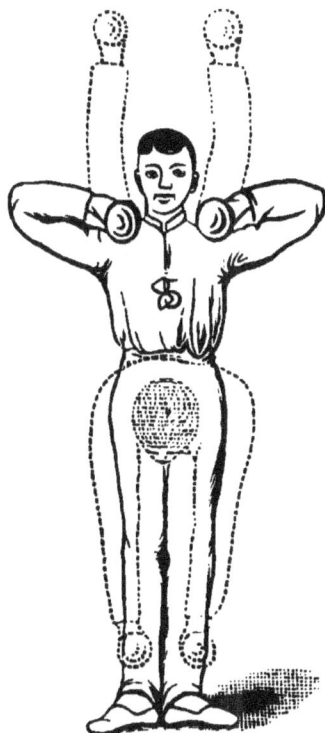

FIG. 8.

count one, bring the bells to the shoulder ; on two, thrust them vertically upward, bells parallel ; on three, return them to the shoulder ; on four, with *knees rigid*, stoop forward, and strike the bells upon the floor ; on count five, return bells to the breast ; on six, thrust upward ; on seven, return bells to the breast ; on eight, strike the floor ; and so continue through twelve counts. [Fig. 8.]

Movement 8. — The bells being at the floor on count twelve, at count one return the bells to the breast,

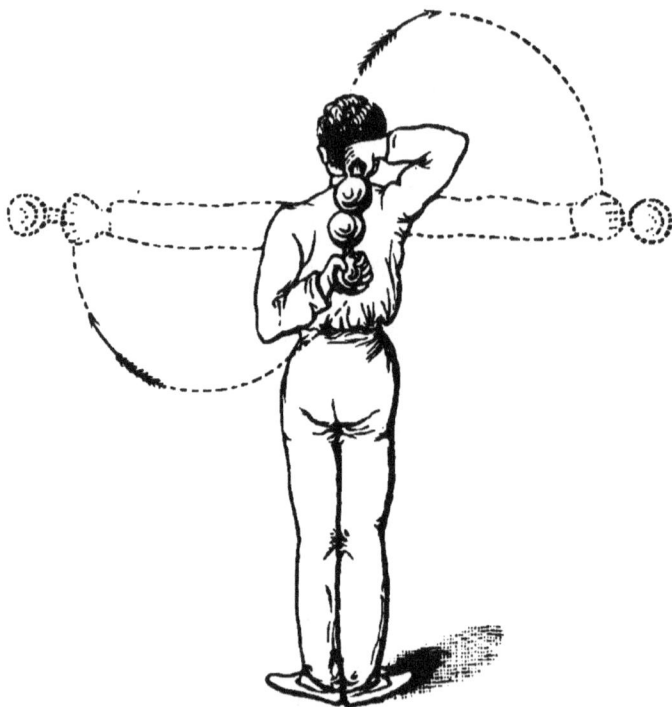

Fig. 9.

and, in so doing, allow the bells to slip through the hand, so that each is held by the end; on count two, extend the arms horizontally outwards, bells horizontal; on count three, put the right bell over the right shoulder, and the left bell under the left shoulder, until the free ends strike behind the body; on count four, bring the bells to the position held at count two; on count five, put the left bell over, and the right bell under, until they strike; and so continue through twelve counts. [Fig. 9.]

Movement 9. — The arms being extended horizontally outwards at count twelve, allow the bells to slip through the hands until they are grasped in the usual manner; on count one, bring the bells to the breast, resting there through count two; on count three, drop the arms to the sides, resting there through count four.

On count one, bend the right elbow, keeping the upper arm fixed, until the bell strikes the shoulder; on count two, drop it back to the side; continuing this movement through eight counts.

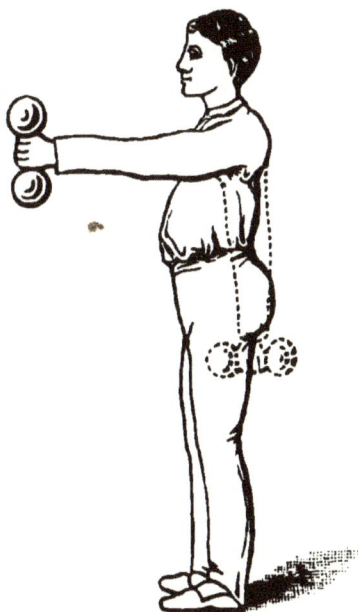

FIG. 10.

The same with the left arm, through eight counts.

The same with the right and left alternately, through eight counts.

The same with the right and left simultaneously, through eight counts.

Movement 10. DIRECTION A. — The bells being at the side at count eight, on count one raise the right arm in a forward direction, so that the bell describes a quarter-circle, thumbs up, elbows stiff ; on count two, return the bell to the side ; and continue the movement thus through eight counts. [See Fig. 10.]

The same with the left, through eight counts.

The same with the right and left alternately, through eight counts.

The same with the right and left simultaneously, through eight counts.

DIRECTION B. — The same as A, except that the arms are raised to the height of the shoulder outward, laterally, bells horizontal.

Movement 11. — Bend the elbow, and raise the right bell to the height of the ear, on count one ; carry the bell

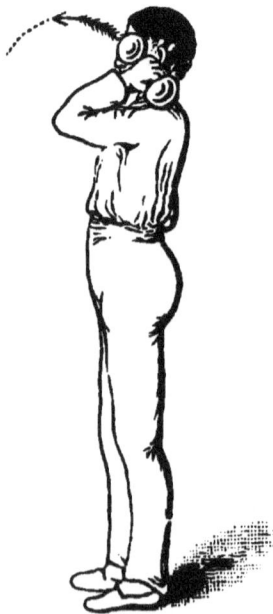

FIG. 11.

back to the side on count two ; and continue the movement thus through eight counts. [Fig. 11.]

The same with the left, through eight counts.

The same with the right and left alternately, through eight counts.

The same with the right and left simultaneously, through eight counts.

Movement 12. DIRECTION A. — With stiff arms describing a semicircle in a horizontal plane, strike the

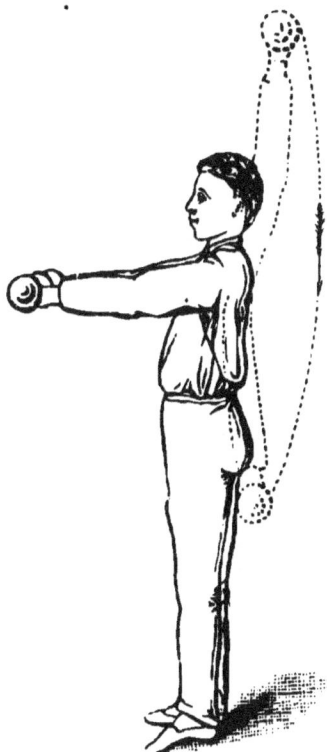

FIG. 12.

bells — on the ends toward the thumbs — together in front; return arms to a horizontal position at the side on count two; strike again on count three; and so continue through twelve counts.

DIRECTION B. — On the count one, with stiff arms describe a semicircle in a vertical plane, and strike the bells — on ends toward the thumbs — together above the head; on count two, return the arms to a horizontal position at the side; and continue thus through twelve counts.

DIRECTION C. — The arms being extended in a horizontal position at the side on count twelve, on count one let the bells describe a semicircle downward, striking together — on the ends toward the little fingers — just behind the body; on count two, strike above the head as before; on count three, behind the body; and so continue through twelve counts. [See Fig. 12.]

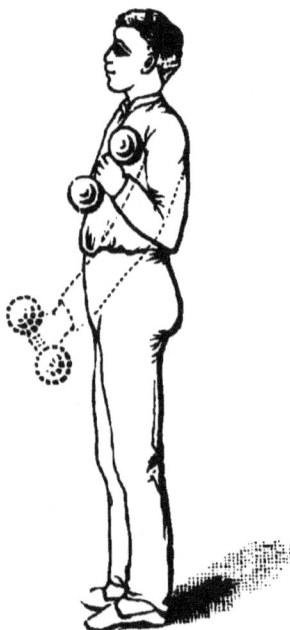

FIG 13.

Movement 13. — The bells being above the head on count twelve, on count one bring them to the breast, and rest there through count two ; on count three, thrust both arms downward and forward, keeping the arms parallel and the bells parallel, the arms making an angle of forty-five degrees with the body ; rest thus through count four ; on count five, return the bells to the breast ; and continue the movement through sixteen counts. [See Fig. 13.]

Movement 14. — On count one, charge the right foot, with a stamp, about sixteen inches to the right, extend

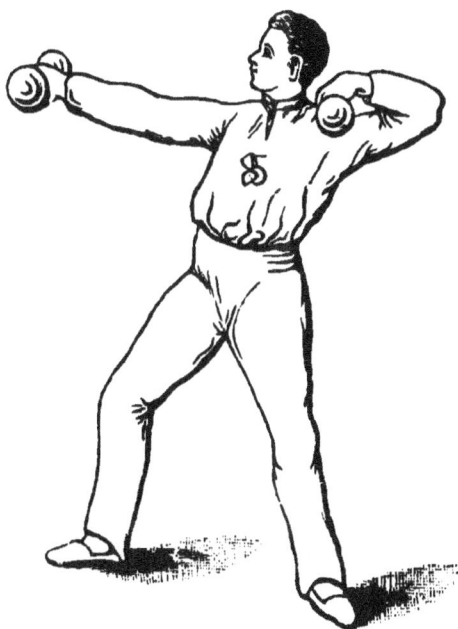

Fig. 14.

the right arm outward horizontally, palm up, bell horizontal ; bring the left bell to the left shoulder, turning the head sharply to the right. On count two, bring the right foot, *without dragging,* to its place beside the left foot, extend left arm to a position like that held by the right, sharply turn the head to the front ; on count three, drop arms, and strike the bells — on the ends toward little fingers — behind the body; on count four, turn the bells, and strike the ends toward the thumbs together behind the body; continue this movement through twelve counts. The same movement toward the left, through twelve counts.

The same alternately to the right and left, through twelve counts.

At count twelve the bells being behind the body, on count one bring both bells to the shoulder, upper arms extended laterally and horizontally; on count two, extend both bells outward horizontally; on counts three and four, strike bells behind the body as above; and continue thus through twelve counts. [See Fig. 14.]

Movement 15. DIRECTION A. — On the count one, charge the right foot with an emphatic stamp in the direction of the right arm of the V, about sixteen inches, turning the body in that direction, and bending the right knee slightly; at the same time bring the bells to the breast. Maintain this position until four counts have been completed. On the count one, forcibly extend the right arm horizontally in the direction faced; on count two, return the right bell to the breast, and extend the left bell; continuing this movement through eight counts. On the count eight, the left arm is extended and the right at the breast; on count one, thrust the right arm outward horizontally, and bring the left to the breast; on count two, bring the right bell to the breast, and thrust the left outward horizontally; continuing thus through eight counts. On count eight, the right bell is brought to the shoulder, the left being extended. On count one, thrust the right bell vertically upward, and bring the left to the shoulder; on two, bring the right bell to the shoulder, and thrust the left upward; continuing thus through eight counts. On count eight, the right bell is brought to the *breast*, the left being thrust upward. On count one, thrust the right bell vertically downward, and bring the left to the breast; on count two, bring the right bell to the breast, and thrust the left downward until the count seven is reached, when the left bell remains at the breast, and the right bell is brought to the breast on count eight. On count one, the body assumes an erect position, the right foot being brought to the side of the left; remain thus through count two. On count three, charge to the left. and remain thus through count four.

DIRECTION B. — Repeat A toward the left The bells being at the breast on the last count eight, on count one let the body become erect, the left foot being brought to the side of the right; remain thus through four counts.

DIRECTION C. — With the body in an erect position facing forward, repeat A.

Movement 16. — The bells being at the breast on the last count eight, on one thrust the right bell forward horizontally, and return it to the breast on count two; on count three, thrust it horizontally outward, and return it to the *shoulder* on count four; on count five, thrust the bell vertically upward, and return it to the *breast* on count six; on count seven, thrust it vertically downward. and return it to the breast on count eight : continuing thus through sixteen counts.

The same with the left bell, through sixteen counts.

The same with the right and left bell alternately. through thirty-two counts.

The same with the right and left simultaneously, through sixteen counts.

Movement 17. — The bells being at the breast on

count sixteen, thrust both horizontally forward on count
one, the bells being perpendicular and two inches apart;
on count two, sweep the arms apart so that each bell
describes a quarter-circle in a horizontal plane; on count
three, return the bells sharply toward each other, as far

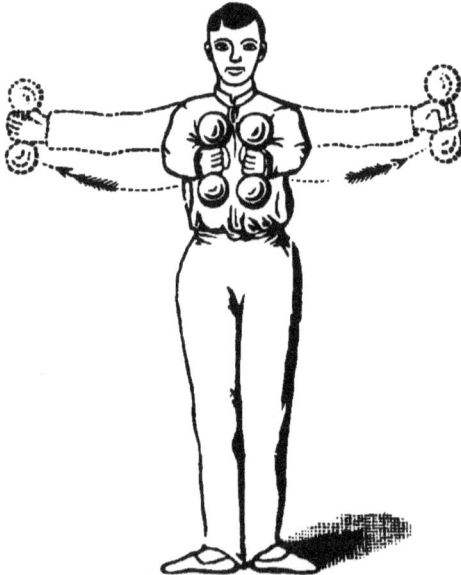

FIG. 15.

as possible without striking; on count four, sweep them
apart again, returning on count five; and continuing thus
through twelve counts. [See Fig. 15.]

Movement 18. — The arms being extended horizontally outward on count twelve, on count one bend the
elbows so as to bring the bells to the shoulders; at the
same time, turn the body in the direction of the right arm
of the V, and charge the right foot in that direction. On
count two, thrust both bells vertically upward, and bring
the right foot to the side of the left; on count three,

return the bells to the shoulder; and, on count four, twisting the bells so that the ends toward the little fingers almost touch, throw the arms outward before the body and downward past the sides, back to the shoulders; continue thus through sixteen counts. [Fig. 16.]

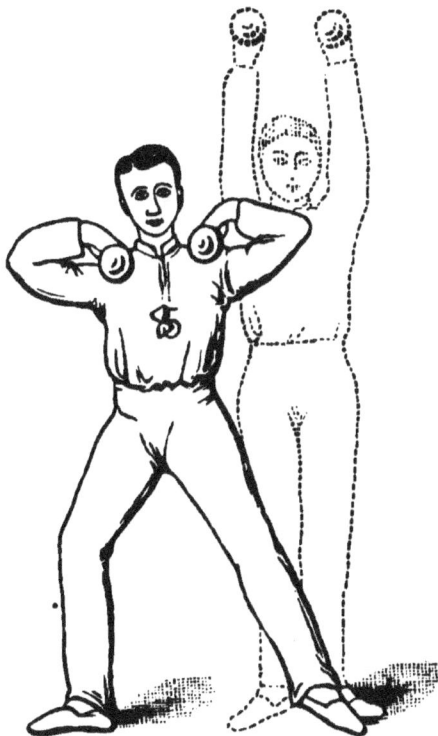

Fig. 16.

The same toward the left, through sixteen counts.

The same toward the right and left alternately, through sixteen counts.

The same motion of the arms directly to the front, with body erect and heels together, through sixteen counts.

Movement 19. DIRECTION A. — On the last count. sixteen, bring the bells together parallel to each other at

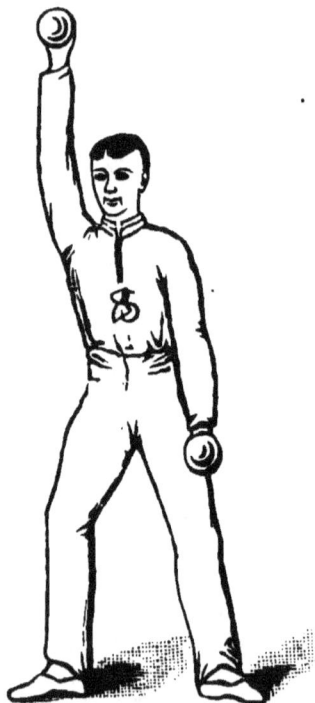

FIG. 17.

the breast, and strike them thus through four counts. On count one, charge the right foot as in Movement 15, thrust the right arm vertically upward, and the left vertically downward; on count two, return the bells to the breast. With foot still advanced, continue the motion of the arms through eight counts, returning the right foot to its place on count eight. [Fig. 17.]

The same to the left, through eight counts.

DIRECTION B. — As at the beginning of this movement, strike the bells through four counts. On count one, charge to the right, thrust right arm up and left arm down, remaining thus through count two. On count three, return the bells to the breast and the foot to its place, remaining thus through count four. On the next four counts, repeat the same to the left; and continue thus alternately toward the right and left, through sixteen counts. Then strike the bells together on the breast as above, through four counts.

Movement 20. — On count one, grasping the bells by the ends, throw the bells over the shoulder until they hang

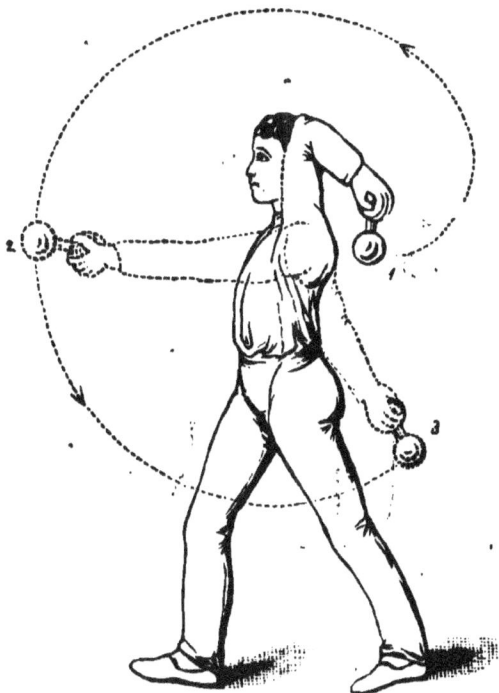

Fig. 18.

almost perpendicularly; at the same time, charge the right foot sixteen inches in the direction of the right arm of the V. On count two, swing the bells forward, allowing

them to describe parallel three-quarter circles as in cut.
The bells should be at 2 on count two, at 3 on count
three, and at 2 again on the return, on count four; on
count three, the foot is placed beside the other. Continue
thus through sixteen counts. [See Fig. 18.]

The same toward the left, through sixteen counts.

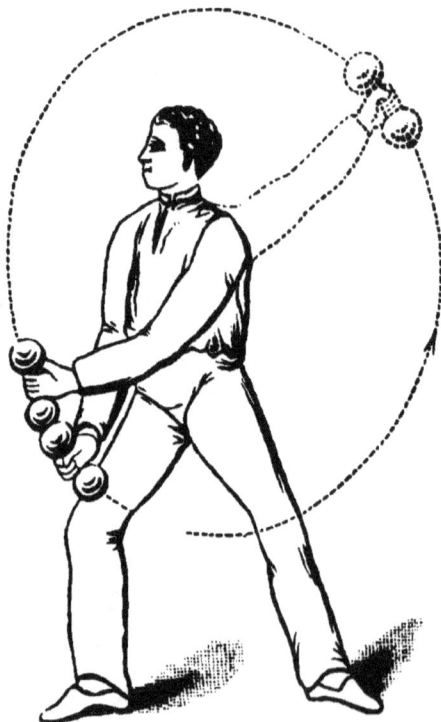

Fig. 19.

The same toward the right and left alternately, through
sixteen counts.

The same directly toward the front, without the charge,
through sixteen counts; on the last count sixteen, let the
bells stop at the side when the arms reach the vertical
position.

Movement 21. — Charging forward with the right foot four inches on each of the next four counts, place the right bell vertically on the right knee; on count one, swing the left arm back in a circle — up and forwards — and strike the bell on every odd count, swinging the arm back on the even counts, through twelve counts; then replace the right foot, stamping four times, and advance the left, repeating the same motions with the bells, after which replace the left foot. [See Fig. 19.]

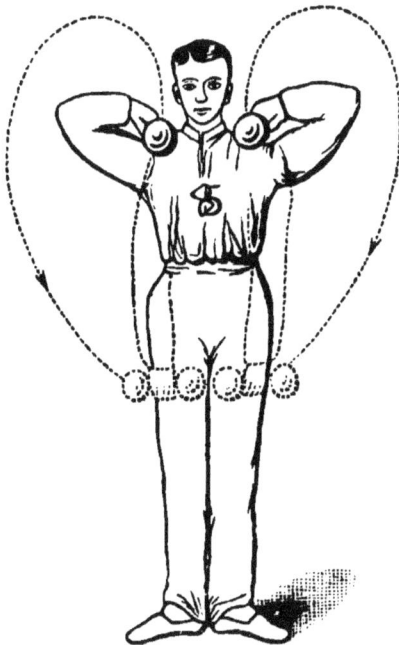

Fig. 20.

Movement 22. — The bells being at the side on the last count, on count one bring each bell to its respective shoulder; on count two, extend the arms horizontally

outward; on count three, strike the bells together — on
the ends toward the little fingers — just in front of.the
body; and, on count four, strike the ends toward the
thumbs together; continuing thus through sixteen counts.
The same, striking behind the body, through sixteen
counts.

The same, striking in front of the body — on the ends
toward the little fingers — on count three, and striking
behind the body — on the ends toward the thumbs — on
count four, through sixteen counts. [See Fig. 20.]

Movement 23. — Repeat Movement 1, Directions A,
B, C, and D, except that on the count seven of D a twist
is made instead of returning to the breast; and the bells
are returned to the breast. and the arms folded promptly,
on the count eight. — which closes the exercise.

THE ANVIL CHORUS: AN EXERCISE IN LIGHT GYMNASTICS.

Tнis Exercise is performed to the music of the Anvil Chorus, from "Il Trovatori," as arranged in the World's Peace Jubilee music of 1872.

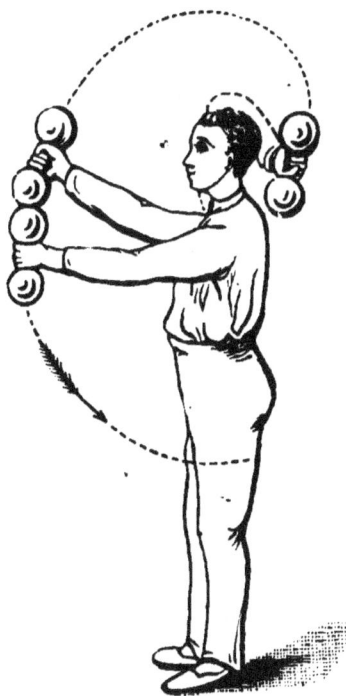

Fɪɢ. 21.

The *Position*, body erect, bells at sides, knuckles in front, is assumed during a prelude, usually beginning at "God of the nations." On fourth count, before "Proudly our banners," etc.. bring right bell to back of neck, thumb down, and left bell to level of eyes in front, arm straight, thumb up. Thus remain through four counts. [Fig. 21.]

No. 1. — Sweep right bell over the head to strike left smartly on the top, on first count, knocking left downward

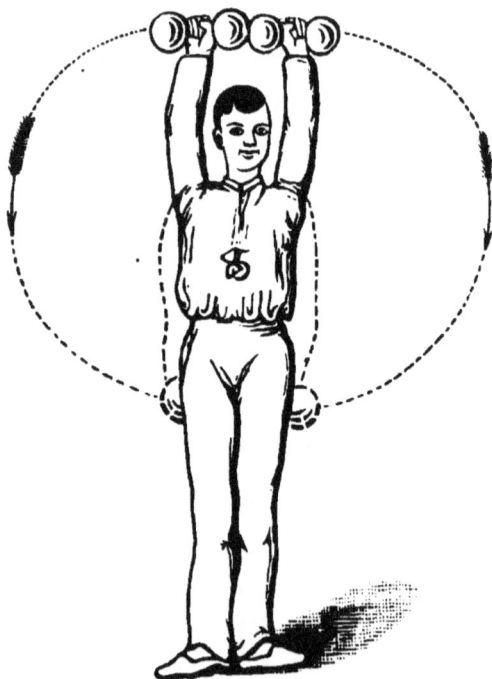

FIG. 22.

and under, arm stiff, to come to back of head on second count, right bell remaining in place of left; on third count, left bell sweeps over, and strikes right, knocking it downward and round to come to back of head on fourth, left bell remaining in place of right; on fifth count, right bell sweeps backward, downward, and under, to strike left bell underneath, and left sweeps over, to come to back of head at sixth count, right bell remaining at level of eyes ; on seventh count, left bell sweeps backwards, downwards, and under, to strike right bell underneath ; and both together sweep upwards, outwards, and downwards, to strike behind the body on the eighth count, little fingers together. [See Fig. 22.]

No. 2. — Strike bells together, arms stiff, thumbs together, above the head, and stamp right foot about eight

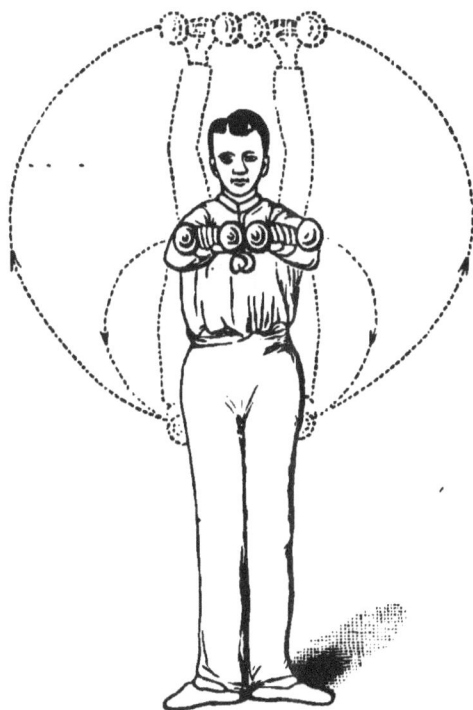

FIG. 23.

inches forward, on first count ; strike downward behind the body, little fingers together, returning foot to position, on second count ; strike above the head as before, stamping left foot, on third ; fourth same as second ; and so on, with alternate feet, through seven counts ; on eighth. come to position assumed at the beginning of No. 1.

No. 3. — Same as No. 1.

No. 4. — With stiff arms, always : on first count, strike bells together at level of eyes in front, thumbs together ; on second, strike downward behind, little fingers together ; on third, strike above head ; on fourth, downward behind ; and so on, through seven counts ; on eighth, come to position assumed at beginning of No. 1.

No. 5. — Same as No. 1.

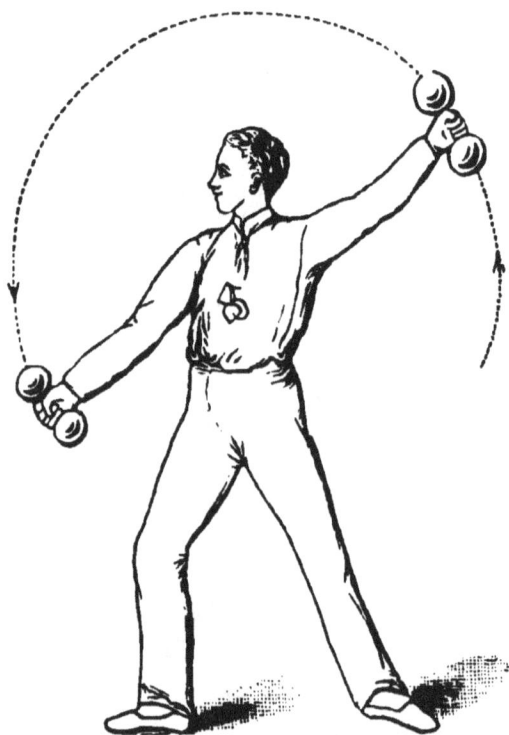

Fig. 24.

No. 6. — Charge laterally to the right, extending right bell over and about six inches above right leg, at same time sweep left bell over to strike right, thumbs together. on first count ; on second, straighten right leg and bend left, keeping feet in place, at same time turning bell once so that the thumb end points in direction in which bell is to go ; sweep it in circle in front of body, arm straight, round to strike right bell on third count, when legs come back into position of first count ; and so on, through seven counts ; on eighth count, come to position assumed at 'beginning of No. 1, springing back with right foot. [Fig. 24.]

No. 7.—Same as No. 1.

No. 8.—Same as No. 6, except charge made to the left, swing right and extend left arm.

No. 9.—Same as No. 1.

No. 10.—Charge to right, extend right bell as before, and sweep left over to strike right on first count; and, keeping legs and feet in position, with stiff arms and full swing strike right bell through the next six counts ; on eighth count, come to position at beginning of No. 1, springing back with right foot.

No. 11.—Same as No. 1.

No. 12.—Same as No. 10, except charge made to left, left arm extended, and right swung in circle. Except, however, on eighth count, coming to erect position, bring bells to chest instead of into position of No. 1, and, at the command "Halt," forcibly bring them to sides, knuckles in front, as at the first.

It will be seen, from the length of this exercise, that the eight measures beginning "Proudly," etc., must be played three times.

It will be both beautiful and beneficial if performed with a *snap*, and every movement vigorously executed. The stiff straight arm must be insisted upon when, according to the nature of the movement, it is not impossible. This specification has been made occasionally through the exercise; being a point most likely to be overlooked and forgotten, and yet of primary importance if either of the above effects would be attained.

TABLE SHOWING THE PRINCIPAL MUSCLES BROUGHT INTO
ACTION BY THE DUMB-BELL EXERCISE OF THE CLASS
OF '85, AMHERST COLLEGE.

THIS exercise is so varied as to bring into action all the
more important muscles of the upper extremity, thorax,
and back, as well as many of those of the lower extremity
and abdomen. It is likewise arranged in such a manner
as to give to each group of muscles an amount of work
proportionate to its relative importance.

In addition to the muscles brought into play by each
particular part of the exercise, the fourteen flexor muscles
of the hand are in constant use in holding the bells firmly
in the grasp.

I. There are, in this exercise, two distinct movements :
1st, rotation of the arm and fore-arm inwards, accompanied by a pronation of the hand ; 2d, rotation of the
arm and fore-arm outwards, with a supination of the hand.
These two movements follow each other in quick succession, and are repeated twenty-four times, six in each of
the positions, *a*, *b*, *c*, and *d*.

1. Rotation of the arm inwards is accomplished by
                    Subscapularis,
assisted by
                    Pectoralis major,
                    Latissimus dorsi,
                    Teres major ;
rotation of the fore-arm, and pronation of the hand, by
                    Pronator radii teres,
                    Pronator quadratus,
                    Flexor carpi radialis,
                    Palmaris longus,
                    Flexor sublimis digitorum.

2. Rotation of the **arm** outwards, by
    Supraspinatus,
    Infraspinatus,
    Teres major ;
rotation of fore-arm outwards, and pronation of hand, by
    Supinator longus,
    Supinator brevis,
    Biceps extensor cubiti,
    Extensor secundi internodii.

II. This may be analyzed into two sets of movements :
1st, a forcible extension of the fore-arm, followed by a
flexion of the same ; 2d, a thrusting of the arm from the
shoulder, in each of the four directions indicated under
a, b, c, and *d.*

    a. 1. Fore-arm extended by
    Triceps,
    Anconeus ;
flexed by
    Biceps,
    Brachialis anticus,
    Pronator radii teres ;
assisted by
    Flexor carpi radialis,
    Flexor sublimis,
    Flexor carpi ulnaris,
    Supinator longus.

    2. Arm extended horizontally forwards by
    Anterior fibres of deltoid,
    Part of pectoralis major,
assisted by
    Biceps,
    Coraco-brachialis ;

depressed to the side by

> Posterior fibres of deltoid,
> Latissimus dorsi,

assisted by

> Subscapularis.

b. 1. Same as *a.*

2. Arm extended horizontally outwards by
> Deltoid,
> Supraspinatus ;

depressed to the side by
> Pectoralis major.
> Latissimus dorsi,
> Subscapularis,

assisted by

> Teres major,
> Teres minor.

c. 1. Same as *a.*

2. Arm raised vertically upwards by
> Deltoid,
> Supraspinatus ;

depressed by the same muscles as in *b.*

d. 1. Same as *a.*

2. The arm lies passive at the side.

III. This is simply a variation of II. As the right arm is raised vertically above the head, the left arm is simultaneously thrust downwards, and *vice versa;* each movement being executed six times.

IV. The bells are now held horizontally outwards. chiefly by the action of the deltoid, during four counts.

V. This motion, as well as the following, brings the

muscles of the shoulder, arm, and fore-arm into most vigorous action.

a. The bells are forcibly drawn down till they meet in front of the body, by the

> Pectoralis major,
> Anterior fibres of deltoid.

Then the arm is twisted, and the hand pronated (see 1), so that the other ends of the bells meet. This latter motion is repeated twelve times.

b. The bells are now drawn behind the body by the

> Latissimus dorsi,
> Teres major,
> Posterior fibres of deltoid :

and the twisting of the bells is repeated in that position, through twelve counts.

c. a and *b* repeated alternately, there being six motions in front, and six behind the body. In all three of these movements, the arm is raised by the

> Deltoid,
> Supraspinatus.

VI. In addition to the muscles of the upper extremity, those of the thigh and leg are used somewhat in retaining the body in the position elsewhere described.

a. Arms raised perpendicularly by

> Deltoid,
> Supraspinatus,

and struck together by the action of that muscle ; then drawn apart by its antagonists, the

> Subscapularis,
> Latissimus dorsi,
> Pectoralis major.

This is repeated four times. Bells are now lowered in

front of the right leg, and struck together; then struck together behind that leg, by the other ends. Finally, they are raised over the head. This is repeated to the left, the left leg being advanced instead of the right.

VII. *a.* **Arms raised perpendicularly upwards, and lowered to the breast, as in II.** *c*; then lowered to the side by extension of fore-arm, as previously described.

b. At the same time, an entirely new set of muscles are brought into play, in drawing the body downwards and forwards; viz., the abdominal muscles, —

> Obliquus externus,
> Obliquus internus,
> Transversalis,
> Rectus abdominis;

assisted by

> Psoas magnus,
> Iliacus,
> Rectus.

This is repeated three times.

VIII. *a.* **Right fore-arm flexed by**

> Biceps,
> Brachialis anticus,
> Pronator radii teres, etc.,

as in II. At the same time, the arm is drawn as far backwards and inwards as possible, chiefly by the

> Deltoid;

left fore-arm flexed as in *a*, and arm drawn backwards and upwards by the

> Latissimus dorsi.

b. Both arms extended to a horizontal position, by an extension of the fore-arm upon the arm, by

Triceps,
Anconeus ;
a lowering of the right arm, by
Subscapularis,
Pectoralis major,
Latissimus dorsi ;
and an elevation of the left, by the
Deltoid.
Repeated six times.

IX. This motion simply exercises the flexors and extensors of the fore-arm. Repeated ten times with each hand. Muscles same as in II. *a* 1.

X. Elbows kept stiff by muscles on back of arms, while the
Deltoid
raises the arms horizontally ; and their own weight, together with the
Latissimus dorsi,
Pectoralis major,
draws them down. Repeated ten times with each arm.

XI. Arm raised forwards and upwards by
Anterior fibres of deltoid,
Part of pectoralis major ;
assisted by
Biceps,
Coraco-brachialis.
Fore-arm flexed as above. Repeated ten times with each arm.

XII. *a.* Elbows rendered stiff by the extensors, and

the arms held in a horizontal position by the deltoid
muscle.   The arm is now drawn forward by the
          Anterior fibres of deltoid,
          Pectoralis major;
then back to a straight line, chiefly by the
          Posterior fibres of deltoid,
          Pectoralis major.

b. Arms in position as above, but raised over the head
until bells strike, by
          Deltoid,
          Supraspinatus.

c. Arms raised as in *b,* and then lowered so that bells
strike below and behind the body, by
          Latissimus dorsi,
          Teres major.

XIII. This is designed to furnish a brief respite, rather
than to exercise actively any set of muscles, and will,
therefore, not be described.

XIV. Right fore-arm extended, and arm raised horizontally outwards, as before described.   Left fore-arm
flexed, and left arm raised horizontally.   Each motion
repeated twelve times with each arm.   At the first four
movements, the right foot is brought forward by flexors
of thighs and extensors of the leg, and, at the end of
each movement, returned to position by the antagonists
of those muscles.   During the next four movements, the
left foot is brought into a similar position.   On the last
four, the body is in its natural position.

XV. This exercise is *essentially* the same as II.   The
arms are alternately thrust in the directions *a, b, c,* and

d, four times with the right foot forward, four times with the left foot forward, and four times with feet together.

XVI. This is another modification of II. Here, each of the four motions *a*, *b*, *c*, and *d*, is performed, in succession, by each hand, and repeated six times by each.

XVII. Same as XII. *a*, with bells *parallel*. Repeated six times.

XVIII. *a*. Arms raised vertically, and fore-arms extended as before ; then arms lowered horizontally outwards, and fore-arms flexed.

b. Arms drawn forwards ninety degrees, and fore-arms extended again to the front. Now, the arm, in describing a circle backwards, is acted upon by all the principal muscles of the arm and shoulder in succession. Repeated twelve times, four times in each of the positions.

XIX. Modification of III. Muscles the same, with the addition of those of the lower extremity used in the charge. Repeated eight times.

XX. *a*. Arms raised to a vertical position by
Deltoid,
Part of pectoralis major.
At this point, the fore-arms are flexed, so that the bells are perpendicular behind.

b. Fore-arms extended, and (with elbows stiff) arms brought forward and downward to the side of the body, by the
Subscapularis.
Pectoralis major,
Latissimus dorsi,

(together with their aids), acting in succession.   Repeated twelve times.

XXI.   The elbow remains stiff, while the arm describes a circle backward.   This brings into play almost all those muscles situated about the shoulder-joint, in different parts of the motion, including all those which can possibly move the arm on the shoulder in any direction.

XXII. Same as V.   Repeated twelve times.

XXIII. Same as I., with *d* repeated *seven* times.

THE MEASURES OF WEIGHT, HEIGHT, CHEST, ARM GIRTH,
LUNG CAPACITY, AND BODY LIFT OF 2,106 DIFFERENT
STUDENTS OF AMHERST COLLEGE, ARRANGED BY AGE.

Age.	Number of observations.	Weight.	Height.	Chest.	Arm.	Lung capacity.	Body lift.
17	330	131.99	66.60	33.87	11.12	224.8	8.58
18	1172	134.07	66.96	35.10	11.36	238.7	10.35
19	1511	135.84	67.30	35.38	11.52	240.3	10.82
20	1358	138.12	67.95	35.52	11.57	248.8	10.97
21	1171	140.00	68.01	35.58	11.69	250.1	10.84
22	807	141.07	68.11	35.98	11.77	250.8	10.92
23	559	141.21	68.31	36.29	11.71	257.0	10.63
24	362	142.42	68.44	37.23	11.74	261.0	10.62
25	216	145.12	68.68	36.66	11.79	263.6	10.11
26	141	144.91	68.82	37.46	11.81	262.5	10.71
27	71	144.40	68.30	36.95	11.84	268.4	10.37
28	30	140.71	68.52	36.28	11.57	269.8	8.51
29	19	142.68	68.09	36.41	11.51	260.5	9.86
30	18	146.50	69.19	36.70	11.61	279.5	7.50

In this table, the average measures of the men of the
ages between seventeen and thirty are given; the second
column shows the weight in pounds and decimals; the
results of height, chest, and arm are given in inches and
hundredths; those of chest capacity, in cubic inches;
and the body-lift means the number of times the indi-
vidual is able to lift the body up to the hands, when
hanging freely suspended above the floor.

A TABLE OF THE BODILY MEASUREMENTS OF THE STUDENTS OF AMHERST COLLEGE, FOR THE YEARS 1881–82, 1883–84, INCLUSIVE, AVERAGED BY YEARS OF AGE.

YEARS OF AGE.	17	18	19	20	21	22	23	24
WEIGHT	59.30	59.70	61.10	61.30	63.20	63.70	63.90	64.70
HEIGHT	1.70	1.70	1.71	1.71	1.72	1.72	1.72	1.72
" Knee	465.00	466.00	469.00	469.00	477.00	478.00	480.00	481.00
" Sitting	887.00	889.00	900.00	901.00	904.00	902.00	902.00	910.00
" Pubes	855.00	857.00	858.00	860.00	863.00	863.00	863.00	867.00
" Navel	1.00	1.00	1.01	1.01	1.02	1.02	1.02	1.02
" Sternum	1.37	1.38	1.39	1.39	1.40	1.40	1.41	1.41
GIRTH, Head	568.00	568.00	568.00	569.00	575.00	575.00	575.00	575.00
" Neck	337.00	341.00	348.00	350.00	354.00	356.00	358.00	356.00
" Chest, full	887.00	903.00	923.00	922.00	925.00	933.00	934.00	942.00
" " repose	853.00	865.00	877.00	883.00	896.00	897.00	899.00	908.00
" Belly	703.00	713.00	714.00	723.00	735.00	736.00	747.00	753.00
" Hips	872.00	875.00	893.00	897.00	900.00	900.00	901.00	901.00
" Thighs	501.00	501.00	512.00	513.00	523.00	523.00	525.00	527.00
" Knees	353.00	354.00	355.00	356.00	357.00	358.00	358.00	358.00
" Calves	337.00	340.00	344.00	346.00	351.00	356.00	357.00	360.00
" Insteps	236.00	237.00	238.00	240.00	243.00	244.00	245.00	247.00
" Right upper arm contracted	275.00	279.00	281.00	284.00	298.00	299.00	301.00	307.00
" Upper arms	242.00	247.00	252.00	253.00	257.00	258.00	261.00	268.00
" Elbows	242.00	243.00	246.00	248.00	251.00	252.00	253.00	254.00
" Fore-arms	251.00	253.00	257.00	261.00	265.00	266.00	266.00	267.00
" Wrists	162.00	162.00	162.00	163.00	166.00	166.00	167.00	167.00
BREADTH, Head	152.00	152.00	153.00	153.00	155.00	155.00	156.00	156.00
" Neck	106.00	106.00	107.00	108.00	109.00	109.00	109.00	109.00
" Shoulders	414.00	423.00	425.00	425.00	435.00	441.00	442.00	442.00
" Waist	247.00	247.00	248.00	248.00	256.00	259.00	259.00	266.00
" Hips	319.00	321.00	325.00	326.00	329.00	320.00	330.00	332.00
" Nipples	188.00	192.00	195.00	197.00	202.00	202.00	202.00	202.00
Shoulder-elbows	362.00	367.00	367.00	369.00	375.00	376.00	376.00	378.00
Elbow-tips	460.00	460.00	460.00	460.00	461.00	462.00	466.00	467.00
LENGTH, Feet	257.00	257.00	258.00	258.00	262.00	262.00	262.00	262.00
Stretch of Arms	1.77	1.77	1.77	1.77	1.80	1.80	1.80	1.80
Horizontal length	1.72	1.72	1.72	1.72	1.73	1.73	1.73	1.73
STRENGTH of Lungs	10.00	13.00	13.50	13.00	12.00	12.00	12.60	12.00
" of Back	132.00	132.00	139.00	146.00	150.00	151.00	156.00	159.00
" Chest, dip	3.60	5.20	5.80	6.20	7.00	7.00	8.20	8.30
" " pull-up	7.60	7.90	8.80	8.90	9.00	9.10	9.10	9.20
" of Legs	160.00	161.00	172.00	180.00	193.00	198.00	199.00	199.00
" of Fore-arm	33.90	34.80	36.10	38.40	40.00	40.10	40.60	40.70
Capacity of Lungs	3.86	3.91	4.03	4.07	4.10	4.20	4.29	4.34
Pilosity	2.10	2.20	2.20	2.30	2.40	2.60	2.70	2.80
NUMBER MEASURED	47.00	100.00	90.00	97.00	50.00	30.00	26.00	11.00
TOTAL	451.00							

The table on page 56 gives the average results of the study of four hundred and sixty-one students, during the past three years, in the more than fifty measures and tests that are applied. They are grouped under the different years of seventeen to twenty-five inclusive; and the results are given in kilograms, metres, and millimetres, except the capacity of lungs, which is in litres, and the chest strength, the unit of which is the bodily weight as raised in a " dip " and a " pull-up."

Such a table cannot show a true ascending and descending grade, on account of its limited data ; but, assuming that the large part of the students approach the normal and healthy standard, their measures will give more than an approximate chart for guiding others of the same ages in the examination and care of themselves.

These data are so obtained as to find out the important facts in relation to the *bones and ligaments*, their size and rate of growth, and at what time of college life they increase the fastest. Some of the *muscles* are measured, especially those of the extremities, to learn the normal size of these parts of the body. Other girths are taken to find out the amount of *skin*, *fat*, and other *protective tissues*. Safe trials of *muscular strength* are employed, not only to test the general condition of muscles, but to know if the different portions of the body are relatively strong, and properly co-ordinated to each other. *Lung tissue* is also tested both in capacity and strength. The stethoscope is used to learn the condition of some of the more important *vital organs*, and lenses to ascertain the refractive power of the *eye*.

BOSTON GYMNASIUM CONSTRUCTION AND SUPPLY COMPANY.

R. J. ROBERTS, President.
Supt. Boston Y.M.C.A. Gymnasium.

A. H. HOWARD, Secretary.
Supt. Dept. Physical Culture, Boston University.

PARFITT BROTHERS, ARCHITECTS.

MANUFACTURERS AND DEALERS IN ALL KINDS OF

Gymnastic Apparatus

BEST SUITED TO THE THOROUGH FURNISHING OF WELL-EQUIPPED

COLLEGE AND ASSOCIATION GYMNASIUMS.

Our architects having made a special study of the construction of Gymnasium Buildings, both in this country and abroad, we are prepared to furnish plans for proposed buildings, and estimates for gymnasium furniture. Those who contemplate putting up Gymnasiums, or fitting up apartments in this line, will find it to their advantage to correspond with us before taking any steps in the matter, addressing all communications to

A. H. HOWARD, Secretary,

No. 9 Ashburton Place, Boston, Mass.

For references, correspond with Dr. E. HITCHCOCK, Amherst College ; R. A. ORR, Secretary Y.M.C.A., Pittsburg, Penn.; Dr. JOHN MASON KNOX, Pres. Lafayette College, Easton, Penn.

1

PRATT'S

ASTRAL OIL

3

F. GROTE & CO.,

IMPORTERS OF AND DEALERS IN

Ivory Goods and Billiard Material.

BUILDERS OF

TEN-PIN ALLEYS AND APPURTENANCES.

Estimates Furnished.

"STANDARD BOWLERS' GUIDE" sent free on application.

114 East 14th Street, New York.

NOTICE!

Amherst College,
Cornell University,
Mass. Inst. of Technology,
University of Notre Dame,

AND OTHERS, ARE LARGE CONSUMERS OF

CHAMPION LOCKS.

These are all brass, four and six tumbler, *new principle, security unequalled.* Every reader is requested to send address for Descriptive Price-List, in which will be found Locks for sundry purposes, including Padlocks, Drawer, Desk, and Closet Locks; also a fine line of *keyless* combination Locks, tin Cash Boxes, etc. Those who enclose a two cent stamp will receive a handy Pocket Tool, made of plated steel. Address

MILLER LOCK CO., Philadelphia.

N.B.—Locks of the brand "Champion" may be bought of any hardware dealer.

4

A STUDY OF THE DRINK QUESTION,

ENTITLED

"THE FOUNDATION OF DEATH."

By AXEL GUSTAFSON. 600 pp. 12mo. RETAIL AND
MAILING PRICE, $2.00.

This book has already been accepted in England as the most complete work on the subject ever published, and one that will be "the Bible of temperance reformers for years to come." It is pronounced the fairest, most exhaustive, freshest, and most original of all the literature on the subject that has yet appeared. It is impartial and careful in its evidence, fair and fearless in its conclusions, and its accuracy is vouched for by the best physiologists and physicians.

In preparation for this work, the author has made exhaustive and impartial researches in the alcohol literature of nearly all countries, having examined, in the various languages, some three thousand works on alcohol and cognate subjects, from a large proportion of which carefully selected quotations are made.

The scope of the work, as to the variety of standpoints from which it is treated, is indicated in the following list of chapters: —

I. Drinking among the Ancients.
   II. The History of the Discovery of Distillation.
  III. Preliminaries to the Study of Modern Drinking.
  IV. Adulteration.
   V. Physiological Results; or, The Effects of Alcohol on the Physical Organs and Functions.
  VI. Pathological Results; or, Diseases caused by Alcohol.
 VII. Moral Results.
VIII. Heredity; or, The Curse entailed on Descendants by Alcohol.
  IX. Therapeutics; or, Alcohol as a Medicine.
   X. Social Results.
  XI. The Origin and Causes of Alcoholism.
 XII. Specious Reasonings concerning the Use of Alcohol.
XIII. What can be done?

GINN, HEATH, & CO., Publishers.

6

THE

Raymond Furnace Manufacturing Co.

OF NEW YORK, AND SOUTH NORWALK (CONN.),

MANUFACTURERS OF

STEAM, AIR, AND WATER

HEATING FURNACES.

ENGINEERING

FOR SETTING FURNACES AND VENTILATION.

DRAINAGE AND PLUMBING

DONE IN ANY PART OF THE COUNTRY.

Send for Illustrated Circular.

Refer, by permission, to Amherst College Officers.